Fit to Fly

Healthy Living Tips for People on The Go

Fit to Fly
Healthy Living Tips for People on The Go
by: Nikki Noya

ISBN: 978-0-359-62155-2
Original Publication: May 1, 2019
Printed in the United States of America.

© 2019 Nikki Noya. All Rights Reserved.

En Pointe Productions, LLC
107 S West Street, #136
Alexandria, VA 22314
www.enpointe.tv

For my family and my clients.

Table of Contents

Health and Wellness

Everywhere I go, people, ask me, "What's in your kitchen? What's your secret?"

The secret is... there is no secret! I know that whatever I put in my body, it affects me, in both good and bad ways. You should love food and learn all the ways nutrition can help you, not hurt you. You should not be afraid to enjoy all the foods you love. I do! Feeling guilty about eating cheese is no way to live. Eating a huge cheese wheel for lunch is no way to live either! Balance, moderation, and attitude are the key ingredients to the true pleasure of eating.

Being smart about food choices is what it's all about. Fresh, organic fruits and vegetables should be the majority of any diet.

Looking good starts on the inside. I want to look and feel great, who doesn't? I want people to be guessing my age for the rest of my life. My lifestyle and nutrition are the secrets to looking my best, from the inside out. Let's face it, if you eat greasy pizza all the time, you will start to look like a greasy pizza! If you are well hydrated and fuel your body with healthy food, you will look fresh, well rested, and your skin will glow.

It's a fact. People who eat well look better. Smart nutrition keeps you young. A diet rich in polyphenols can protect against those nasty free radicals that want to damage and age your skin. Polyphenols antioxidants are found in things like blueberries, spinach, olive oil, and walnuts. I want to have all of my organs with me for the rest of my life, so I feed my machine with the fuel it needs to keep going and going and going.

So, what do I actually eat on a daily basis? Well, today for example, I had a huge glass of water to get things going. Then, I had coffee with soymilk (I'm lactose intolerant). After that, I made a smoothie with frozen peaches and raspberries, ground flaxseed, banana, and lots of blueberries. I like to add something called "green machine" which is a vitamin powder that has tons of vitamins and minerals in it. I share it with my family. I'll also have a little cup of oatmeal. Irish steel cut oatmeal is the best. I like to put natural peanut butter or cinnamon and honey on mine.

I wake up starving and consider breakfast very important. A lot of my wellness and nutrition clients do not share my love of breakfast and that's ok. If you don't want to eat first thing in the morning, that's alright. Just don't wait too long to eat that by lunchtime you are starving and the only thing that will satisfy your hunger is a double cheeseburger. And fries. And a Coke. And a cookie...

Eating a healthy diet when you're traveling isn't easy - especially if you're going for a long car ride. Typical road trip fare includes fast food, microwave-ready service station options, bags of chips and lots of sodas, but it is possible to navigate your way around the junk food and maintain your healthy diet.

Even if you're seriously strained for time and you absolutely can't resist the airport restaurants, staying hydrated will do absolute wonders for your travel day.

Drinking water will help with many of the obstacles that often arise throughout your travels. It can enhance your mood (a sense of humor is important when your flight is delayed), prevent headaches, aid in digestion and help with appetite control.

Someone is Fit to fly when they plan ahead. Here are my simple tricks to make traveling comfortable, easy and so when you land at your destination you are ready to go!

Hydration and Why It's Important

Water is essential for life. Approximately 60 percent of the human body is made of water. The brain and heart are composed of 73 percent water while the lungs are about 83 percent. Water is simple and, one hopes, pure. We often take it for granted until we are in a situation where fresh drinking water is scarce or unavailable.

The knowledgeable traveler is mindful of the body's water requirements. Air travel and travel in general create an increased need for hydration. Not only do travelers experience physiological changes related to an increase in altitude and cabin pressure, they are also exposed to low moisture levels. Aircraft cabin humidity levels are unnaturally low, about 5–10 percent, creating an environment with less humidity than the Sahara Desert!

Dehydration also exaggerates jet lag. Symptoms of dehydration may include dry or chapped skin, increased wrinkles, dry eyes, thirst, tiredness, dry mouth, headache, constipation, dizziness or lightheadedness. Severe dehydration may result in low blood pressure, rapid heartbeat, extreme thirst, dry skin, loss of skin elasticity, confusion, and fever. Research shows adequate water intake may prevent deep vein thrombosis (blood clots in your legs), pulmonary embolism (blood clot in your lungs) or heart attacks, especially when traveling.

One of the most important habits to cultivate

is drinking two 8-ounce glasses of warm or room-temperature water upon awakening. Drinking water in the morning proves an effective energy booster.

To experience the positive benefits of adequate hydration, tune into your thirst cues. Many people actually eat when they are thirsty instead of providing their body with water. To encourage water intake, fill a bottle or pitcher with your daily water requirement in the morning and drink it throughout the day. Set it on the counter where you will see it and be reminded to drink.

While traveling and during flight, drink at least 8 ounces of water per hour and avoid drinking alcohol, which dehydrates your body. The body uses water to process other beverages we consume. Increased water intake may send you to the bathroom more frequently, but think of it as exercise. There is conflicting evidence whether or not caffeine-containing beverages have a diuretic effect, but excessive intake can cause dehydration.

How much water is enough? On average, adults need six to 10 cups (8-ounce cups) of water a day. Determine if you are drinking enough by noting the color of your urine output. If it is clear or slightly yellow, you are well-hydrated. Some individuals with medical conditions such as kidney failure or congestive heart failure cannot tolerate the recommended level of water intake. Consult your physician regarding your personal health needs.

Drink as much water as possible in the days leading up to your trip. Consider bringing a refillable bottle on your trip and filling it at your gate. Many gates now provide stations where you can fill a reusable bottle in order to prevent the plastic from going to landfills. Others haven't caught on to this trend, so you may have to buy a bottle.

Benefits of Staying Hydrated

Water Increases Your Energy Levels

Traveling is fun, there is no doubt about it, but it's also tiring. Moving from time zone to time zone can throw your body's internal clock all out of whack. This can tend to make you tired, zapping your energy. In addition, if you are participating in an activity, you need extra hydration as proper hydration can improve your endurance and reduce fatigue according to the Journal of Athletic Training. Suffice it to say, that drinking adequate amounts of water will help improve your energy levels.

It Prevents Illnesses and Flushes Toxins

Proper hydration is a key component of properly functioning kidneys. The kidneys, of course, serve the primary purpose of removing waste from your body naturally. In addition, a body that is properly hydrated will tend to restore nutrients quicker, preventing illnesses. Therefore, when you don't get enough water, your body's natural waste removal system gets a little backed up and can even stop working altogether if dehydration sets in.

Water Keeps Skin Moist And Healthy

Everyone wants to look good while traveling. After all, those pictures are going to be around forever! However, there is nothing attractive about dry, flaky skin, which can occur when you don't drink enough water. Thankfully, you can keep your skin moist and healthy and even reduce the appearance of fine wrinkles and lines simply by drinking enough water according to The American Academy of Dermatology.

It Improves Your Overall Mood

Vacation or traveling is no time be in a bad mood. After all, you want to take in all the adventures your vacation has to offer. When you fail to make hydration important enough, though, your body can begin to get dehydrated. Unfortunately, this can cause headaches along with moodiness according to the Journal of Nutrition.

Water Improves Cognitive Function

Have you ever found yourself reaching for a sugary treat in the late afternoon when you need a mental boost? Instead, you might try a tall glass of water. That's right, according to a study found in the Frontiers in Human Neuroscience, simply drinking a glass of water can enhance your brain's cognitive ability.

You Are What You Wear

Oh, travel days. It's so easy to just throw on an outfit and head to the airport while rushing for a flight. Dressing appropriately for air travel means knowing what will keep you comfortable on the plane—and given the cramped seats and various temperature changes on flights, this isn't always easy.

Air travel is often an assemblage of various disparate micro-climates, from the sweat-inducing sunny tarmac to the arctic air-conditioned cabin during flight. So fight discomfort with plenty of layers. You can wear a washable cotton scarf that's a large enough to double as a wrap when it's particularly chilly. Wraps, cardigans, sweatshirts, vests, and light jackets are perfect. You can even fold or roll soft items, like cotton jackets, and use them as makeshift pillows during flight. Plus, the more layers you pile on your body, the less you need to pack in your luggage.

Layers that help you regulate temperature while flying also come in very handy when traveling through various (actual) climates. And for travelers hitting the road during shoulder season when the weather is particularly unpredictable, layers are key for optimal comfort.

Maintain in-flight comfort and cleanliness by wearing breathable fabrics – materials like cotton or linen. Fabrics that don't allow air to circulate will hold sweat on the skin, likely making you feel dirtier faster and probably necessitating a good spin in the washing machine upon landing. Natural fabrics are great, but moisture-wicking manmade fabrics are suitable options as well.

We've all been there. You packed a dress for a special event, only to unpack and discover it's a wrinkled mess. Or you thought jeans would be a good idea on the plane, and now they're cutting off your circulation midflight. From discomfort to wrinkles and funky odors, the fabrics you choose can make or break your travel days. Avoid silks, nylon, leather, rubber, and more generally, clothes made from a synthetic material.

It's best to wear extremely comfortable, mostly flat shoes on the plane – think of your poor feet after hours or even days of sitting, standing, and walking en route to your destination. You'll also want to select comfortable shoes that are easy to slip on and off when passing through airport security.

Deep Vein Thrombosis (DTV) is a danger on flights,

where travelers stuck in cramped seats for long periods of time are at greater risk for developing blood clots. To reduce the risk of getting DVT, the University of Washington Medical Center recommends avoiding "tight clothing, nylons, or socks (especially the type that are too tight at the top and/or leave marks on your skin) that might restrict blood flow through veins." So leave your skinny jeans at home and opt for less restrictive garments like loose-fitting dresses or more relaxed-or wide-leg pants.

Food for Thought – Pack Your Own Food

If you have ever traveled by air, you know that food options are becoming more and more limited. Some airlines do not offer food at all, apart from a packet of pretzels. Others offer food for purchase, including snack boxes, pre-made sandwiches, and fruit and cheese plates. Unless you are able to travel in business or first class, you have few options.

You can buy food at the airport and take it onto your airplane, but if you find yourself short of time or don't care for any of the airport's food offerings, you are out of luck. If you have food allergies or follow a specific diet, you are even worse off. Airport food is expensive, too.

Your best bet, if you want to save money and eat the foods you like, is to prepare your own travel meals. Here are some tips for making and carrying food for your next airplane flight.

The Transportation Security Administration prohibits all liquids and gels in containers larger than 100 milliliters (just over three ounces) in carry-on baggage. Liquids and gels may be brought in these smaller quantities, provided that all such containers fit into one quart, zip-close plastic bag. "Liquids and gels" include peanut butter, jelly, frosting, pudding, hummus, applesauce, cream cheese, ketchup, dips, and other soft or pourable food items. The only exceptions are baby food, baby milk, juice for infants, and liquid medicine (with a written prescription).

This prohibition extends to ice packs, whether they

are gel or liquid. Keeping cold foods cold may be difficult on long flights. Flight attendants may not want to give you ice from their freezer to use in your cooler, so you will need to find ways to keep your food cold or pack items that can be kept at room temperature.

The TSA carefully scrutinizes food brought through the security checkpoint, so you need to pack some non-"gel" food to get by in case your "gel" food is confiscated. Pack food in clear containers or bags whenever possible.

Sandwiches, wraps, and salads are easy to carry and eat on an airplane. You can make your own or purchase them from your favorite grocery store or restaurant. Be sure to carry them in secure containers to prevent leaks.

Fruit travels well. Dried fruits are portable and delicious. Bananas, oranges, tangerines, grapes, and apples are easy to carry and eat. Be sure to wash your fruit at home.

Granola bars, energy bars, and crackers are easy to carry. Sliced cheese is tasty, but must be kept cold or eaten within four hours after coming out of the refrigerator. If you like to snack, consider packing vegetable chips or other junk food alternatives.

You can buy beverages in the airport terminal once you have passed through security. You will be offered a beverage on your flight unless the weather is poor or the flight is extremely short.

To save money, take an empty bottle through the security checkpoint and fill it before you board. You can bring individual-sized flavor packets with you.

Why Pack Your Own Food?

There are lots of reasons as to why you might want to pack food for a trip.

✓ If you have dietary restrictions or allergies, as I do, it can supplement your meals until you can find an appropriate alternative.

✓ You might be a long term traveler who wants to carry food to cook to save money on meals out.

✓ You also might be a picky eater who wants to be sure of what they're eating. Or you're afraid of getting sick.

✓ Packing your own food prevents hanger, which affects even the best of us.

Traveling With Kids

If you think managing a baby is a tough task, then imagine the challenge you would face while traveling with a baby in tow. You may be unsure about the kind of food to carry while travelling with baby and toddler. To keep your baby's hunger satiated and her mood happy, you will have to be innovative and use a wee bit of common sense.

Make travelling with kids a little easier and less stressful by packing them a box of these tasty and healthy snacks.

Travelling with kids can be stressful enough, but when you add food into the equation it's a total minefield! The right travel snacks can make or break a journey. Believe me, the last place you want to be stuck with a hangry child is on an airplane or in the car on the motorway.

There's no shortage of sugary treats in airports, on planes and in service stations. So when packing snacks, stick with healthier options and that way you know the kids will be getting a balance of treats versus the nutritious stuff.

Don't pack anything that is going to be difficult for the kids to open and eat by themselves. Really messy food should be avoided too. It will inevitably end up all over them and probably your car too! Small packets of snacks are ideal as they are easy to eat with little mess.

To boost the nutritional content of their snack packs make sure you add in some veggies. Carrots, cucumber, celery and peppers can all be cut in advance and will last several hours in an airtight lunchbox.

Travelling with your baby should be special for you and your baby. Feeding your baby or toddler during a trip should not cause any stress. All you require is effort and loads of patience, so the journey becomes enjoyable with food and feeding times being the least of your worries.

Sleep Happens

Sleep plays a vital role in good health and well-being throughout your life. Getting enough quality sleep at the right times can help protect your mental health, physical health, quality of life, and safety.

The way you feel while you're awake depends in part on what happens while you're sleeping. During sleep, your body is working to support healthy brain function and maintain your physical health. In children and teens, sleep also helps support growth and development.

The damage from sleep deficiency can occur in an instant (such as a car crash), or it can harm you over time. For example, ongoing sleep deficiency can raise your risk for some chronic health problems. It also can affect how well you think, react, work, learn, and get along with others.

Sleep plays an important role in your physical health. For example, sleep is involved in healing and repair of your heart and blood vessels. Ongoing sleep deficiency is linked to an increased risk of heart disease, kidney disease, high blood pressure, diabetes, and stroke.

Sleep deficiency also increases the risk of obesity. For example, one study of teenagers showed that with each hour of sleep lost, the odds of becoming obese went up. Sleep deficiency increases the risk of obesity in other age groups as well.

Sleep helps maintain a healthy balance of the

hormones that make you feel hungry (ghrelin) or full (leptin). When you don't get enough sleep, your level of ghrelin goes up and your level of leptin goes down. This makes you feel hungrier than when you're well-rested.

Sleep also affects how your body reacts to insulin, the hormone that controls your blood glucose (sugar) level. Sleep deficiency results in a higher than normal blood sugar level, which may increase your risk for diabetes.

Sleep also supports healthy growth and development. Deep sleep triggers the body to release the hormone that promotes normal growth in children and teens. This hormone also boosts muscle mass and helps repair cells and tissues in children, teens, and adults. Sleep also plays a role in puberty and fertility.

Your immune system relies on sleep to stay healthy. This system defends your body against foreign or harmful substances. Ongoing sleep deficiency can change the way in which your immune system responds. For example, if you're sleep deficient, you may have trouble fighting common infections.

Sleep, like nutrition and physical activity, is critical to our health, and when we don't get enough, we sacrifice more than just a good night's sleep.

Exercises on the Road

Sightseeing, singalongs and snack stops can be fun while road-tripping, but sitting for long periods of time can wreak havoc on your body and health. Over time, excessive sitting can not only have a negative impact on your posture but also contribute to an increased risk of cancer, heart disease and even premature death, according to a recent meta-analysis published in the Annals of Internal Medicine.

When we are seated, much of our anterior musculature (internal shoulder rotators, hip flexors) becomes tight and shortened, while the opposite side of our body becomes inactive and lengthened. This effect can lead to cramping, lower back pain, poor posture and even more significant health risks, such as deep-vein thrombosis. It's important to incorporate regular intervals of activity that help stretch the front of the body and activate the back of the body.

To combat those physical maladies, here are some moves that target the three main areas of the body that get tight when you choose to drive: hip flexors, lower back, and your mind.

This might be hard to do in a moving vehicle, so wait until you get to a rest stop.

Simple Meditation

Stand tall, hands at heart center. Close your eyes and simply think "I am inhaling...I am exhaling." Let the breath be fluid and easy. Do it for as long as you can (while still keeping to your travel schedule!), but even if you only take a few moments here, it's beneficial. You'll get back in the car much more peaceful and ready to take on whatever traffic the road has in store for you.

Forward Fold Hang

Stand with feet inner-hips-width apart, and gently fold your upper body over your legs. Place a slight bend in your knees to make a shelf for your torso, and hold for 5-10 breaths to let the whole spine release. Option to grab for opposite elbows and sway from side to side. Option to take this one with legs crossed for an outer-hip stretch.

Full-Body Stretch

Stand tall, root your feet into the ground, take a big breath in, and sweep your arms all the out to the sides, then up. On your exhale, bring your hands to heart center. Repeat 3-5 times, focusing on lengthening the front and sides of your body on the inhales, and grounding on the exhales. Make every breath bigger and more energizing than the last.

If your hotel doesn't have a gym, is your training routine doomed? Not really. If your hotel has a gym, great!

The best exercise while traveling is always walking. Little things like taking the stairs, skipping the moving walkway and walking to your gate instead of people mover are easy ways to get moving. Bring the right shoes. When you have the right shoes, exploring and taking the long way are easy. Don't make the "my feet hurt" excuse.

Business Trip Blues

✓ Cocktails have calories – But a little red wine can be very good for you. Stick to the two glass max rule and your skin will thank you too.

✓ Get away from processed foods – Why would you want to put those chemicals in your body? - this is hard to do on the road but remember... The more color, the better – Think of bright blueberries, eggplant, spinach, peppers. Colors mean vitamins and minerals... make your plate as colorful as possible!

✓ Turn off the TV and sit down – Distracted eating means overeating.

✓ Insure – Take a multi-vitamin. Keep your bases covered. Make sure you take it with food!

Exercises on the Plane

Long haul flights can be really tough on you if you don't approach them the right way. To keep your cramped body from getting too stiff at 35,000 feet, here are seven exercises you can do on the plane to loosen up. After a few hours in a plane, there's a good chance your limbs and muscles will need to move.

Sitting down for long periods of time can you make you more susceptible to Deep Vein Thrombosis (DVT) - poor blood circulation that causes blood clots to form.

Things like making circles with your feet, pulling your knees up, rolling your neck, and taking an occasional stroll down the aisle (when the seat belt light is off, of course). It may seem like these exercises are really simple, but you might be surprised what a little movement can do for you in the long run.

Here are a few exercises that will help:

Neck Roll

If your head is unsupported in an upright position, or you find yourself sleeping with your head in an awkward position, this can cause neck ache (especially if the aeroplane cabin has cold air flowing through it!)

Make sure you stretch your sternocleidomastoid muscle (this runs down the side of the neck from beneath the earlobe to the top of the shoulder). You can do this by tipping your head to one side and applying light pressure from the top of the head to bring your ear closer to your shoulder (keep your chin forward and your shoulders level).

High Knees From Your Seat

High knees are a great way to stretch out and get your blood flowing. You can replicate this same movement without getting up out of your seat. Bend forward slightly and put your hands around one of your knees. Then slowly pull that knee towards your chest. You should feel a slight stretch in your glutes. Hold for 10 seconds and then alternate knees. Do five repetitions on each side and then go back to watching that rom-com.

Calf Raises

Blood-clots commonly form in the lower extremities. It very important to increase the flow of blood by flexing your calf muscles. Hold onto a seat back or another sturdy object for support. Stand with your feet hip-distance apart and slowly rise up onto your toes. Hold for a second or two, then slowly lower down. Repeat 10 to 20 times.

Here is the perfect five step program:

Step 1:

- ✓ With your hands clasped together, raise your arms slowly above your head
- ✓ Stretch them up towards the celling, rather than backwards
- ✓ Slowly turn your palms to the ceiling as you stretch
- ✓ Relax and then repeat three times

Step 2:

- ✓ With your hands clasped together, pull your left knee slowly up to your chest
- ✓ Hold for a count of eight, then release and relax

- ✓ Now do the same with your right knee, then with both knees together
- ✓ Repeat the whole sequence four times

Step 3:

- ✓ Lift one foot off the ground
- ✓ Rotate the ankle gently and slowly 10 times to the left, then 10 times to the right
- ✓ Now, flex the foot up and down 10 times
- ✓ Relax, then repeat with the other foot
- ✓ Repeat the whole sequence three times

Step 4:

- ✓ Turn your head 90 degrees to one side, by rotating your neck slowly and gently
- ✓ Don't overstretch or move too quickly
- ✓ Keep your shoulders down and relaxed
- ✓ Now turn your head to the other side
- ✓ Repeat four times on each side

Step 5:

✓ Sit back in your seat - relaxed but upright

✓ Now close your eyes, take a deep breath and as you breathe out, think 'relax'

✓ Be aware of all your muscles and try to relax any of them that feel tense

✓ Repeat this exercise three or four times

Exercises You Can Do Anywhere

You don't need a gym to get moving. Your body was made to move, and these simple exercises can be done first thing in the morning while you are getting ready. Plus they will get you ready for a full day of sight seeing, visiting museums, hiking, snorkeling – whatever is on your agenda for fun.

Squats

The Squat is a lower body exercise. You can do the bodyweight version, without added resistance (also called Bodyweight Squat or Air Squat), or with weights such as a barbell (Front Squat and Back Squat are variations of the Barbell Squat).

The Squat exercise mainly targets the thighs (quadriceps & hamstrings) and the glutes. However, core strength & stability, ankle mobility, back muscles, calves, and other factors play an important role when you are doing this exercise.

Lunges

The lunge is probably one of the most versatile exercises in our strength training tool box. It gives you the biggest bang for your buck.

Some of the benefits of performing lunges are:

- ✓ strengthening the glutes, quadriceps and hamstrings
- ✓ improves posture
- ✓ develops core strength and stability
- ✓ improves balance and coordination

The lunge is one of our primal patterns. This is

a movement that is stored in our brains from early development.

A longer stride in the lunge will work the glutes, hamstrings and posterior chain more. A short stride lunge will emphasize the quadriceps. Personally, I prefer the long stridden lunge as this is also safer for the knee.

Pushups

Push-ups are one of the best exercises around. The reason push ups are one of the best exercise is the countless variations available of the exercise.

You can also vary the difficulty of the exercise by how wide apart you position your feet. Feet wide apart creates a more stable base, thus making the exercise easier. Feet close together destabilizes your base and more muscles engage to keep your balance.

Once you have mastered feet close together, raise one foot off the ground to make it even more difficult.

You could even switch how you position your hands. Start out with thumbs facing in, with fingers forward. You could also try staggered hand position or one hand on a weighted ball. Theses variations will target your chest and shoulders differently.

Tricep Dips

The purpose and intent of the triceps dip exercise is to strengthen the upper body, and increase the range of motion of the body – as a whole. This particular exercise has been proven to be highly effective in building up the strength of the triceps, the shoulders, and the arms.

There are many health benefits associated with the triceps dip exercise. First, you only need your own body weight to perform the exercise and a sturdy chair. As you start engaging in the exercise, you will find that tension is eliminated from the shoulders.

Planks

Planking has become increasingly popular for core strengthening, and for good reason: it works – in large part because it engages multiple muscle groups simultaneously.

The plank is one of the best exercises for core conditioning but it also works your glutes and hamstrings, supports proper posture, and improves balance.

You can perform the plank in many different directions: front, side, and reverse—each direction engages different sets of muscles for all-around toning and strengthening. The front-facing plank engages the following upper and lower body areas: abdominals, lower back, chest, shoulders, upper trapezius, and neck, biceps, triceps, glutes, thighs, and calves. Side planking is particularly effective for training your obliques, which really helps stabilize your spine, while the reverse plank places the focus on your glutes, hamstrings, abs, and lower back. It can be difficult at first. Don't give up and keep increasing your hold day by day.

Fitness Apps to use While Traveling

Travelling is an amazing way to escape routine and shake up your life, but it can take its toll on your fitness. If you're a long-term or frequent traveller, not having control of when and where you exercise, what you're eating, and how much sleep you get, takes a big toll on your health.

If you're trying to get in shape, especially while traveling, apps can be extremely helpful. When you're on the road and not keeping a normal schedule, apps can provide workout routines, track your progress and, most of all, keep you accountable.

Exploring while you are traveling is the best way to keep up with your wellness program, learn about different cultures, eat amazing food and maybe make new friends! While I am traveling these are the apps I love:

Map My Run

When running apps were first introduced, the fact there existed only a few made the decision process of who to use much easier. Today, the entire fitness app industry has proliferated and there are now dozens of options, many of which have similar features — this makes picking one especially difficult. With so many to select from, how do you know which might provide the specific functionality you're looking for?

MapMyRun offers the ability to track activities like road running, trail running, walking, cycling, mountain biking, interval training, and a slew of others. It offers a blank starter map which allows you to leapfrog from location to location to design a fully customized route. You can also surf through other user-generated maps or even redo previous runs you've recorded live.

Once your workout is complete, MapMyRun generates a chart which tracks your pace and speed changes throughout the run, broken down into custom splits, and highlights where the hills and inclines were located. You can also view detailed graphs of your heart rate and see how much time you spent across the various cardio zones. Amazing right?

AllTrails

AllTrails opening screen presents you with a list of nearby trails and a thumbnail summary of the name, rating, and location. You can switch to map view to see them pinned to a map around your location. It's easy to find trails elsewhere because you can search in any location.

AllTrails is one of the most popular hiking apps available. The free version allows you to create your own trails with GPS tracking, photos and text, and save or share them with others. The annual membership gives you access to the premium version, the advantages of a partnership with National Geographic Maps, and the ability to print and edit maps.

Maps Me

Maps Me is quickly becoming the go-to offline app/maps app for travel.

The main benefit of using Maps Me is that the maps app is completely offline. This means you can download map data in a custom compressed formation that is updated 1 – 2 times per month. All of the maps are stored locally on your device so there is no need for an internet connection once you have downloaded the map.

This can be incredibly handy when you don't have access to a cell tower, are traveling in a different country, use paper maps, or simply don't want to be tethered to needing data. When we travel, we always preload the maps to our phones so we always have access to our location and local resources.

Map Me can be used for everything: driving, hiking, biking, and walking. I can't imagine traveling without it.

Scan and Translate

One of the most useful innovations, instant camera translation has taken translation apps to the next level because they use your phone's camera to analyze foreign text and translate it right in front of your eyes.

If you travel frequently, you could use an app

that can read street signs in a foreign country through live camera translation. If you buy products from overseas, you could translate the instruction manual via the instant translation. Imagine being in a fancy restaurant and you can't read the menu items that are in a different language, those days are history now with instant camera translation.

It saves some time by not having you to type it all in, especially for large chunks of text. There are a lot of reasons why it's extremely handy to have this on your phone.

HighFive

This is an easy to use video conferencing app. In our travels, you do not have to lose contact with your family and friends at home. I'm sure you'd be excited to show them all that you are experiencing in the new city. No better way to achieve this than with the Highfive app. Here, video conferencing is made easy.

Recipes

Nikki's No-Fuss Famous Turkey Chili Recipe

Ingredients:

- ✓ 1 or 2 packs of chili seasoning like McCormicks
- ✓ 2 lbs ground turkey
- ✓ 1 large can diced tomatoes
- ✓ 1 large can kidney beans
- ✓ 1 large can pinto beans
- ✓ 1 red onion (if you like)
- ✓ shredded lowfat cheese- any kind
- ✓ a LITTLE beer-yes trust me Corona or Presidente work best
- ✓ 2 limes
- ✓ Lots of garlic powder, onion powder, lemon pepper, mixed up salt
- ✓ (I never really measure anything, I go on taste)

Preparation:

- ✓ Drain Beans
- ✓ Brown the turkey in big skillet
- ✓ Dice onion and throw in with the turkey
- ✓ In big pot bring to boil beans and tomatoes
- ✓ Add chili seasoning to turkey and mix really well... add everything together in the pot. Roll limes on counter then squeeze juice into pot. (Little trick)
- ✓ Add a little cheese and beer to chili (yes trust me still)
- ✓ Turn down heat and simmer
- ✓ Add spices as you like
- ✓ Let sit for awhile and enjoy with a little low-fat sour cream or salsa!

Nikki's Quick Ground Turkey Dinner Salad

Ingredients:

- ✓ 1 lb. ground turkey
- ✓ olive oil
- ✓ Worchester sauce
- ✓ green olives
- ✓ capers
- ✓ cilantro
- ✓ chopped onion
- ✓ baby bella mushrooms
- ✓ chopped green peppers
- ✓ pine nuts
- ✓ arugula
- ✓ brown rice
- ✓ lemon pepper

- ✓ arugula

- ✓ brown rice

Preparation:

- ✓ Bring a small to medium sized pot of water to boil for your rice. In a medium skillet on medium heat, quickly caramelize your onion adding your ground turkey a little at a time mixing in with the wooden spoon. Keep an eye on it, turning every few minutes with the spoon, add a little water as needed to keep it from charring on bottom of pan and keep the juices going. I usually toss in the peppers and mushrooms for the last five minutes or so to warm them up, but not over cook them, I like my vegetables a little firm.

✓ When turkey is nicely done, add capers, olives, cilantro, Worchester sauce and pine nuts. In big bowl combine turkey and onion, mushroom, pepper mix stir with lots of love.

✓ serve over arugula and brown rice

Savory Chicken Tacos And Guacamole

Ingredients:

- ✓ 1 lb. ground chicken
- ✓ watercress
- ✓ I package baby bella mushrooms
- ✓ 1 chopped leek
- ✓ minced garlic
- ✓ 1 package low sodium taco seasoning
- ✓ low fat sour cream, if you like
- ✓ Crumbled low fat goat cheese
- ✓ endive or iceberg lettuce

For Guacamole:

- ✓ 2 ripe avocados
- ✓ cilantro
- ✓ lime
- ✓ garlic salt and pepper

Preparation:

- ✓ In a small pan, sauté mushrooms, leeks and garlic until desired brown chicken on medium heat in large pan gradually add taco seasoning with water to browned chicken Combine vegetables to chicken and add any remaining seasoning.
- ✓ While chicken is browning: mash avocadoes, chop cilantro, squeeze in lime and add garlic salt and pepper to taste. Admire beauty of guacamole and don't forget to smile.
- ✓ Scoop chicken and vegetable mix into lettuce leaf or endive leaf and finish with a sprinkle of goat cheese and low fat sour cream if you like, or simply add guacamole and enjoy!

Nikki's Quick+Easy Beauty Salad

Ingredients:

- ✓ Watercress
- ✓ mixed greens
- ✓ 1 avocado
- ✓ 1/3 cup walnuts
- ✓ 1/2 apple
- ✓ 1/ 3 cup feta cheese
- ✓ Lemon pepper

Salad dressing:

- ✓ 1/3 cup olive oil
- ✓ 1/3 cup Dijon mustard
- ✓ Pepper
- ✓ A pinch of onion or garlic salt
- ✓ In plastic container, shake shake shake dressing ingredients until desired consistency
- ✓ mix salad ingredients together and enjoy

About The Author
Nikki Noya

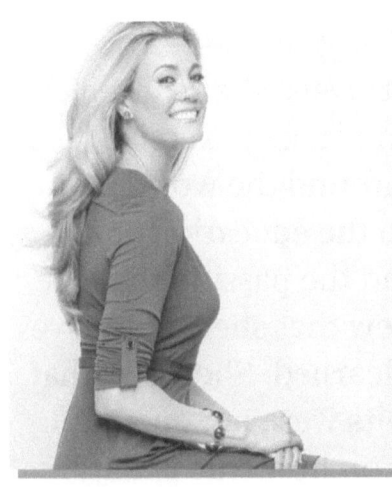

Exercise has always been an integral part of Nikki Noya's life. A sports fanatic and enthusiast, she found her early passion in the pool, where she achieved countless accolades and awards during her high school years, including four Junior Olympic Championship medals, Junior Lifeguard of the Year in Newport Beach, Calif., Student of the Year at Our Lady Queen of Angels School, and Commissioner for Women's Athletics at Mater Dei High School in California.After watching professional volleyball player Gabrielle Reece, Nikki became inspired and decided to try the sport. After just one practice, she was captivated and loved the feeling of being part of a team. By her sophomore year of high school, she had made the varsity team, been quickly named Team Captain, and received the Scholar Athlete Award. Under Nikki's leadership, her team ranked third in the nation. Her remarkable volleyball abilities led to a full scholarship to the University of Rhode Island, where her team became the Atlantic 10 Conference Champions.

Through her extensive travels, she realized how obesity, poor nutrition and lack of exercise affected the lives of so many around the world and across the United States. With the education and tools that she had acquired and the passion that she felt for helping others, she knew that she had to give back and share what she had learned. She knew that exercise and smart eating habits were not enough; she had to educate her clients on how true beauty starts from within.

This is where the Nikki Noya brand was born. As a Wellness Coach, she strives to empower clients to achieve vibrancy, energy, radiance, and beautiful health. Through fitness, nutrition and balance, clients become their best, feel their best, and look their best. They discover the anti-aging benefits of nurturing nutrition and learn how food and movement can be their greatest beauty tools and ultimate allies.

Now Nikki serves as co-host of the nationally syndicated travel and lifestyle talk show "The Jet Set," she also is Vice President of Dress for Success and started a spin-off called "Vets for Success." She is seated on two boards: Becky's Fund and the University of Rhode Island Harrington School Advisory. She and her husband has also created the Noya Fields Family Fund, a scholarship program for female students at various colleges. To date, the NFFF has provided over $500,000 worth of scholarships to deserving students.

For more information visit: NikkiNoya.com

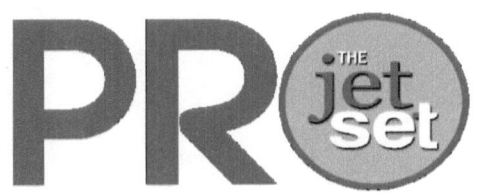